PREFACE

Dedicated to my parents who kept me safe during and throughout my Epilepsy journey. Also reminding me I can still do most things and to not be scared to try. They made sure I was receiving the best care. They advocated for me when I know it was a scary time for them to watch there child grow up with medical road blocks. My brother was also by my side growing up and even though he is younger he was very protective of me.

Also to my amazing husband and life partner he has taught me true love exist. He continues to keep me safe and gave me the gift as a bonus Mom. I've been lucky enough to raise my now two stepsons over the past almost 20 years.

Lastly my Grandfather WWII vet I was honored to be a part of his life. Taught me the power of what strength is. Reminded to me never to be afraid, to always be kind and don't let fear stop you from trying anything.

"So you have Epilepsy, do have any questions?" The Doctor looked at her and asked waiting for her response? She was to scared to talk. She felt numb and confused on the inside.

She remained quiet while her Mom spoke up and tried to talk to the Doctor for her. The Doctor immediately spoke over her Mother and said she has a voice and she needs to answer the question.

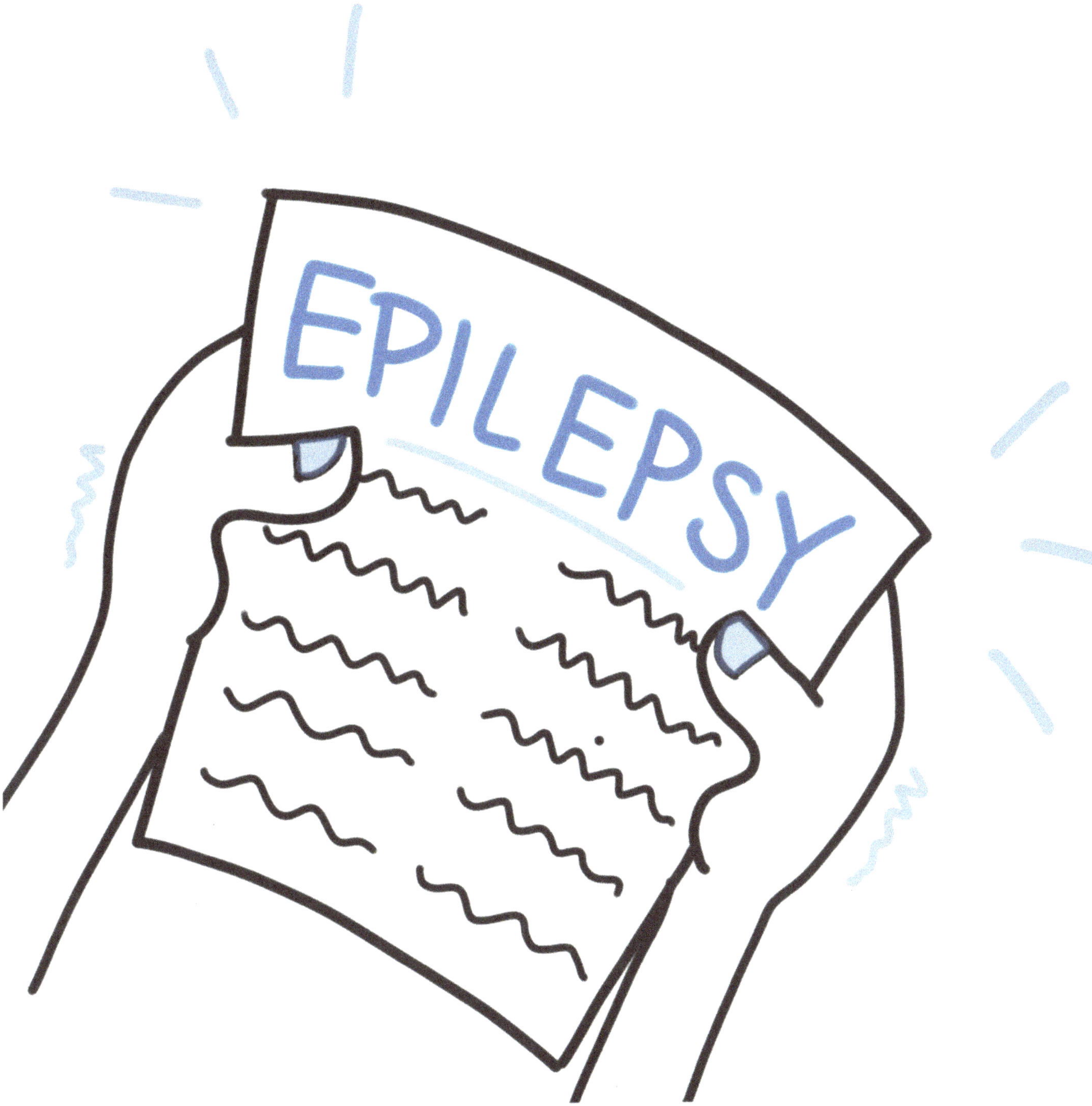
EPILEPSY

She was only thirteen and to scared to answer the doctor. Epilepsy? That sounds like a scary word she thought. The Doctor said to both her and Mother she will be fine just read the brochure. The Doctor handed the brochure to her Mother and he left the exam room.

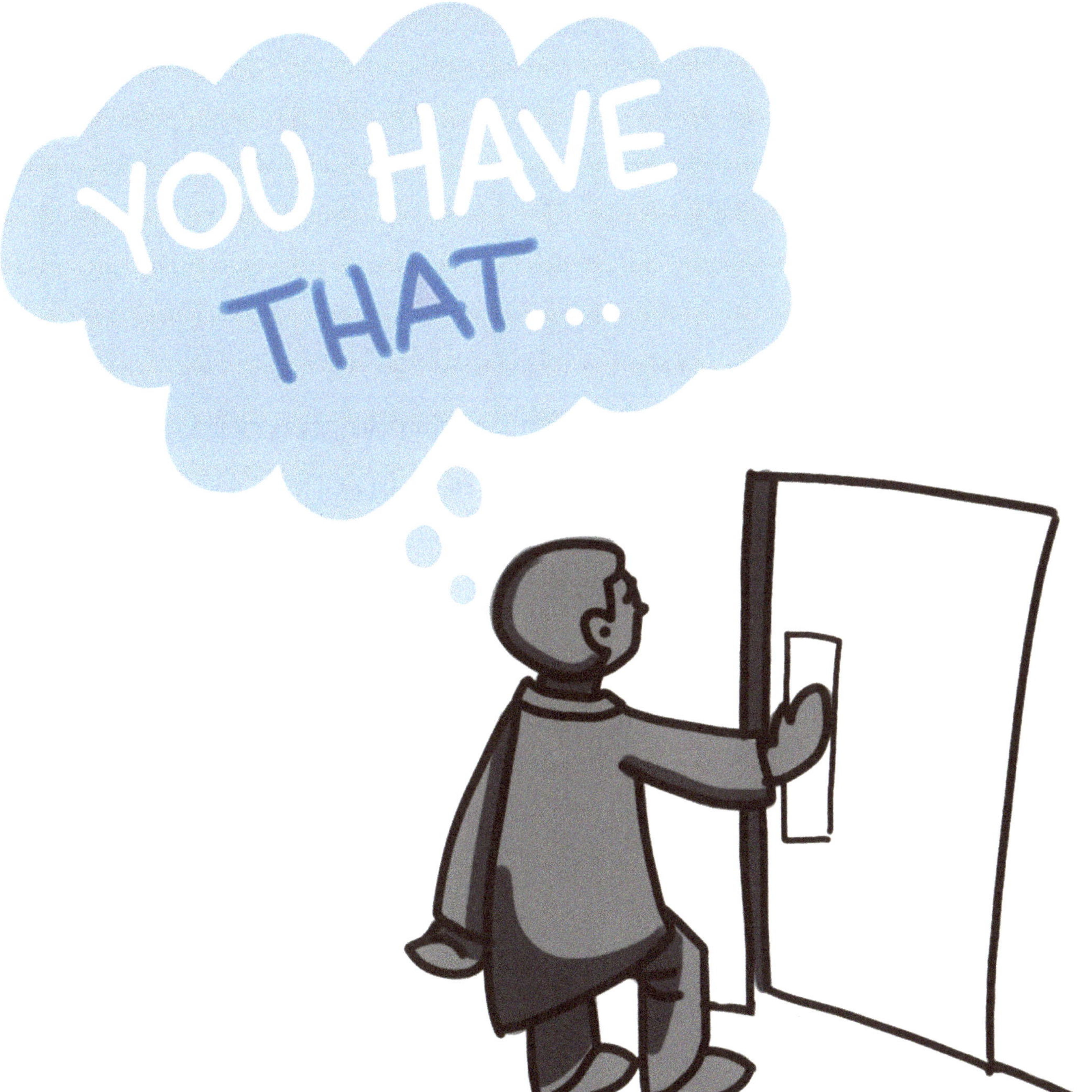
YOU HAVE
THAT...

With all these new restrictions on her life what would she be able to do she thought. She was able to continue dance thankfully. No contact sports was just the beginning of the list she would never be allowed to do.

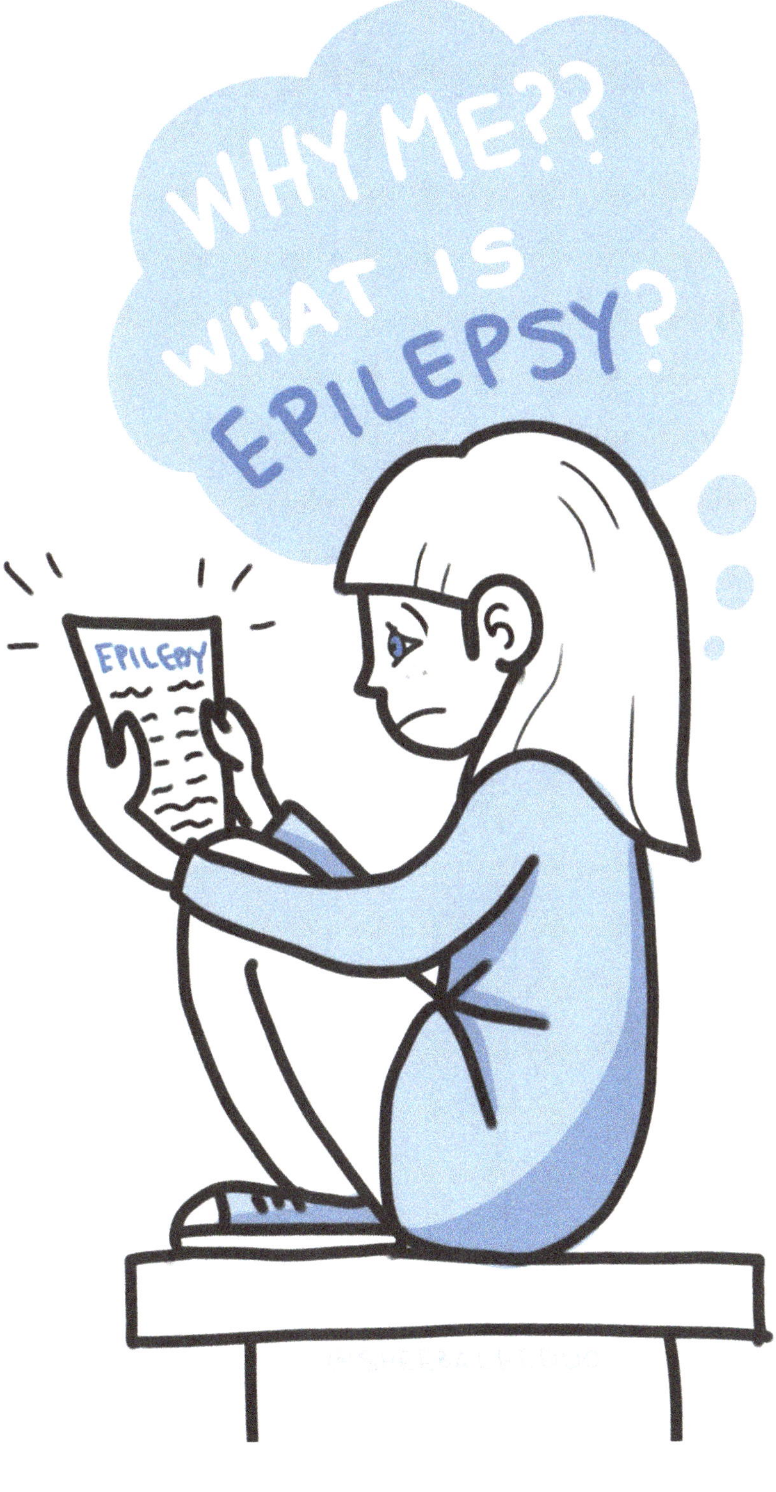
WHY ME??
WHAT IS
EPILEPSY?
EPILEPSY

Even though she was given all these new life changes and restrictions. Her brain started to wonder what can she do… Despite all the negative new life changes she couldn't control. This voice kept saying you'll be fine and made her wonder what she instead could do.

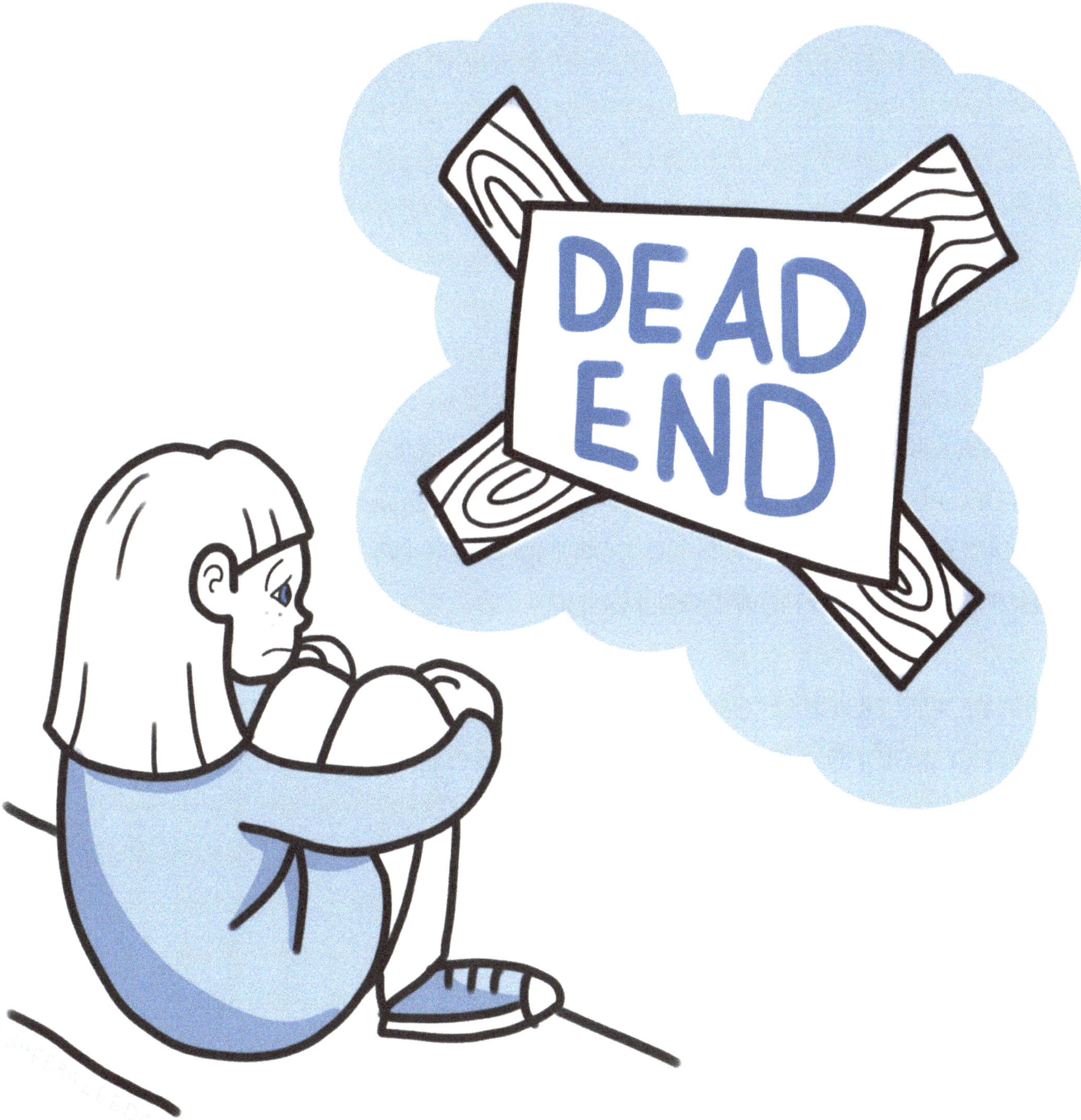
DEAD
END

She would realize going to school was going to be different. It didn't take long with gaining weight after starting her new medication. She would be coming back to school with a new diagnosis and a new body type.

She would quickly realize how her body had changed after gaining weight. She would be mocked and bullied for it.

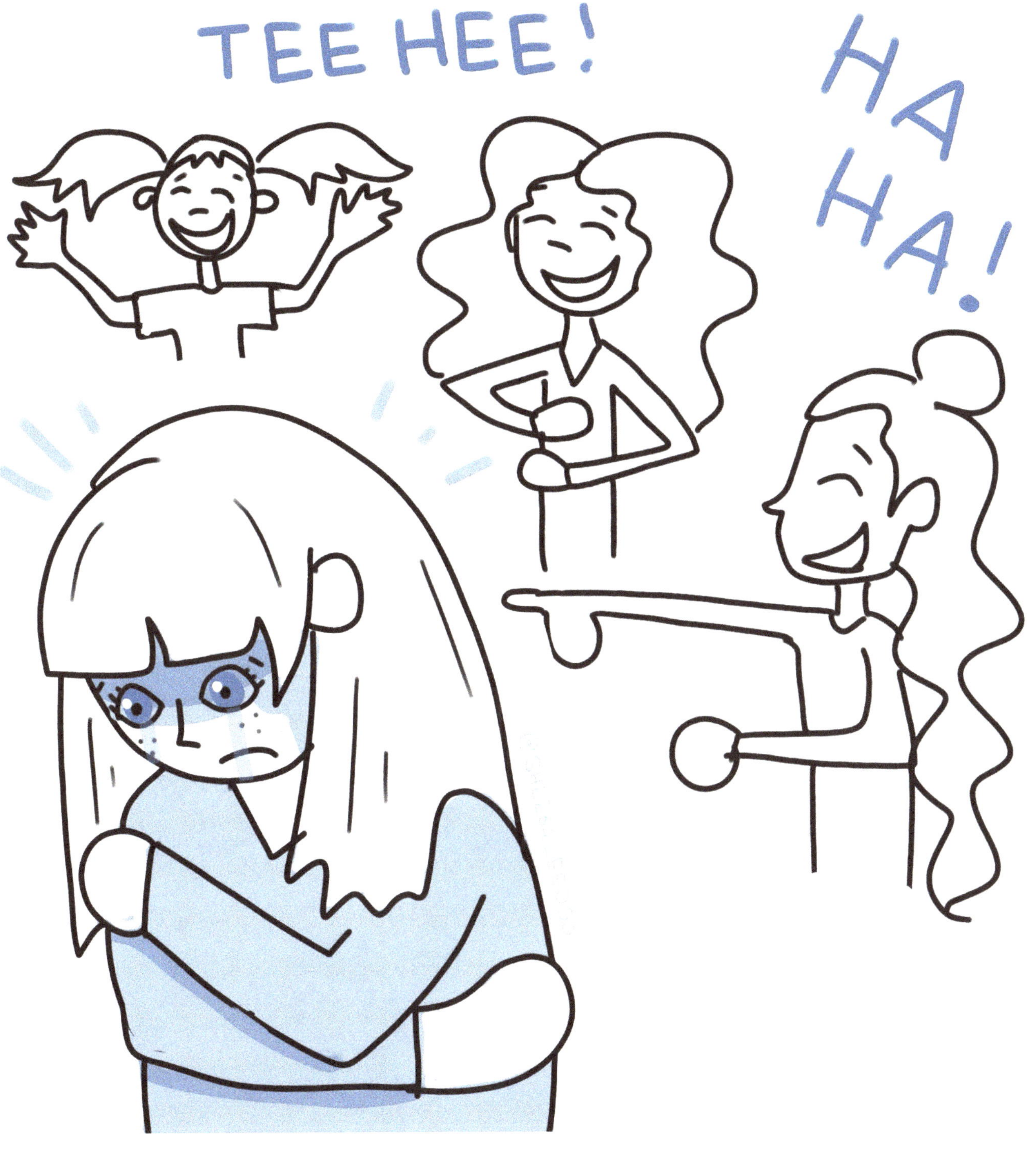
TEE HEE!
HA HA!

She could still go traveling and camping with her family. She and her family would go to almost every KOA they could. She could still go fishing with her brother and Dad.

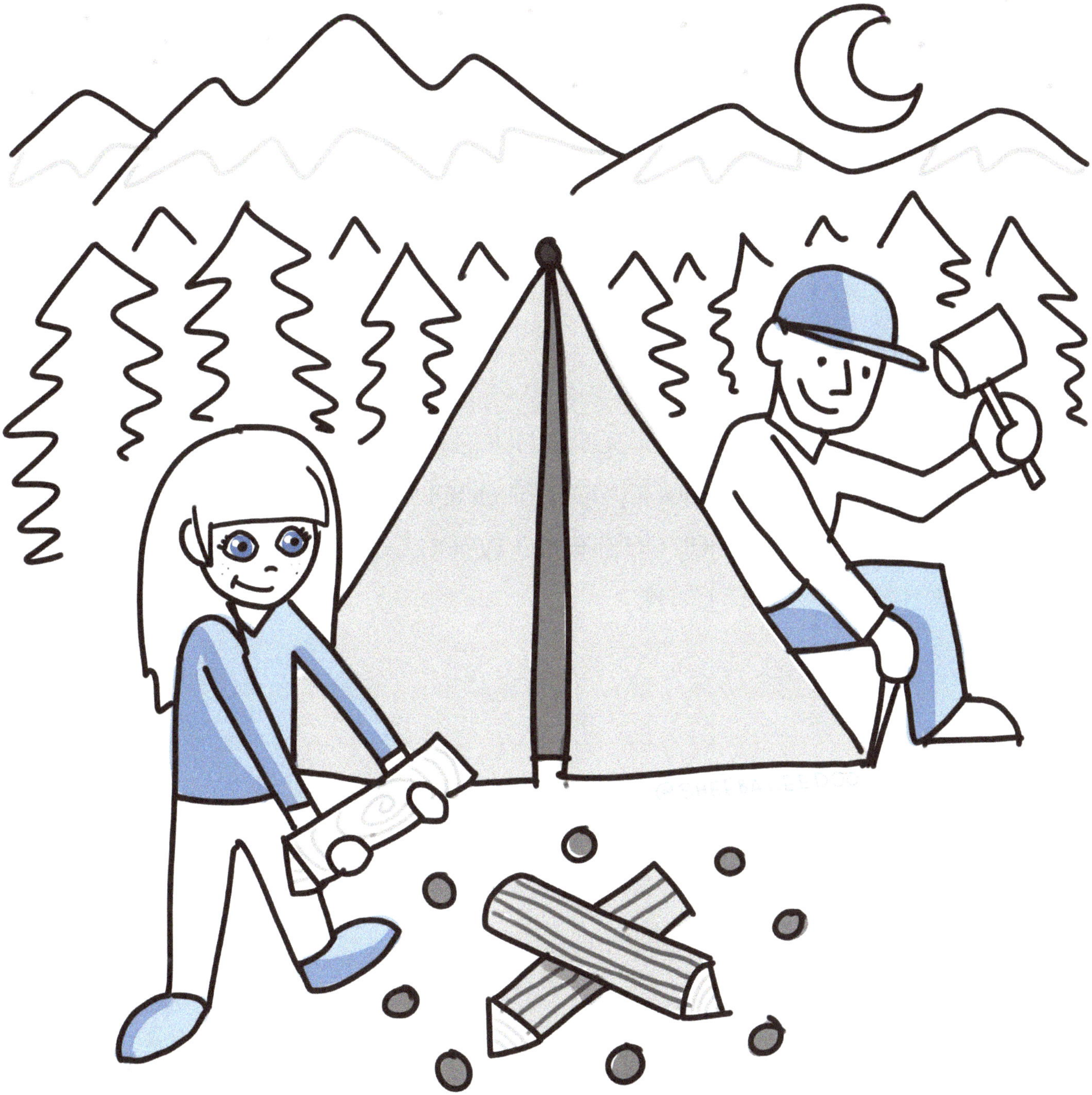

She could still go for motorcycle rides with with her Dad. She would learn at a very young age all about motorcycles. That would later turn into her desire to want to learn how to ride and have a bike of her own.

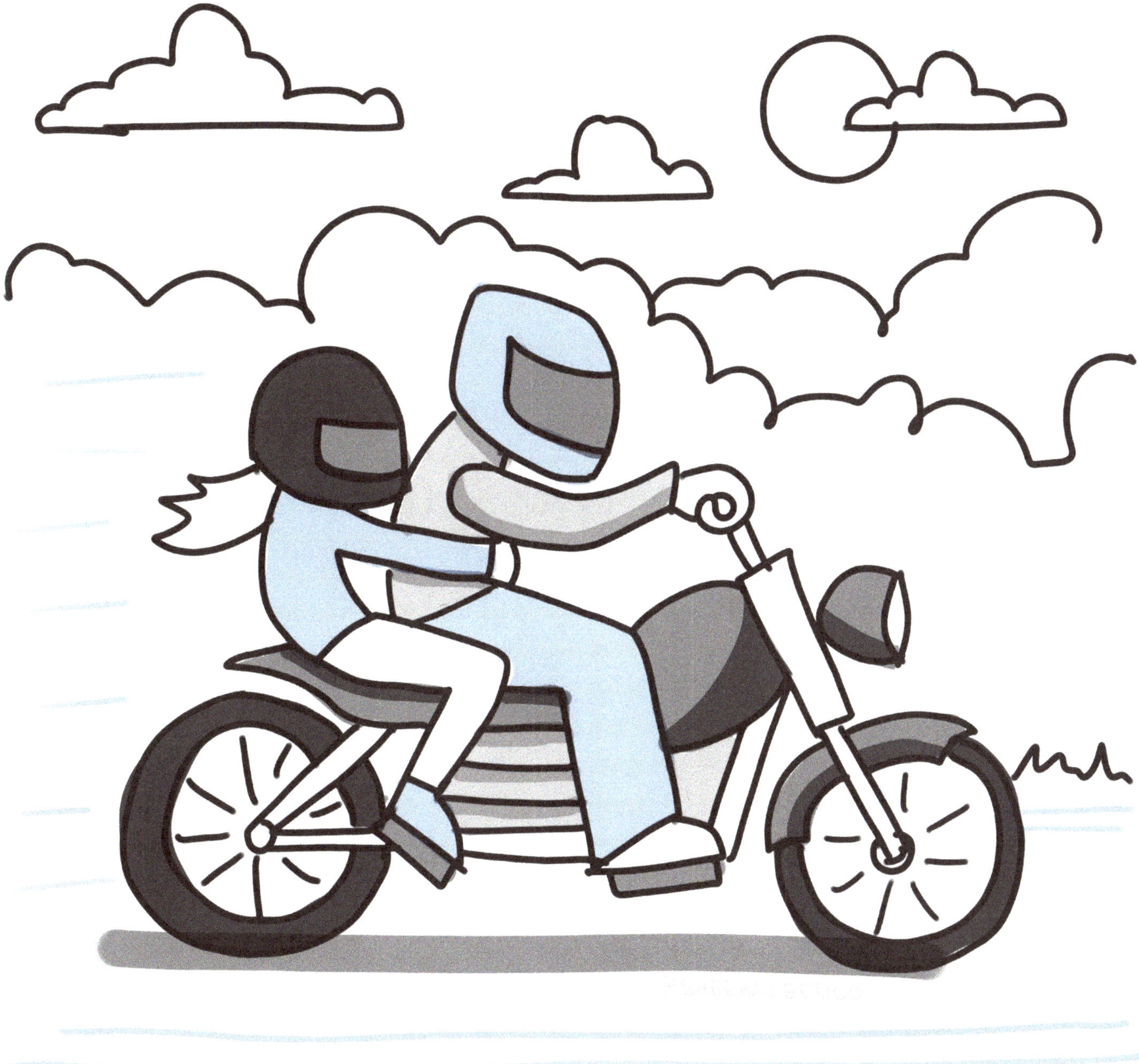

She could still dance which continued for almost 14 years. She could still sing in choir which she did for 10 years. She could try color guard and basketball cheer leading that she only survived 1 year.

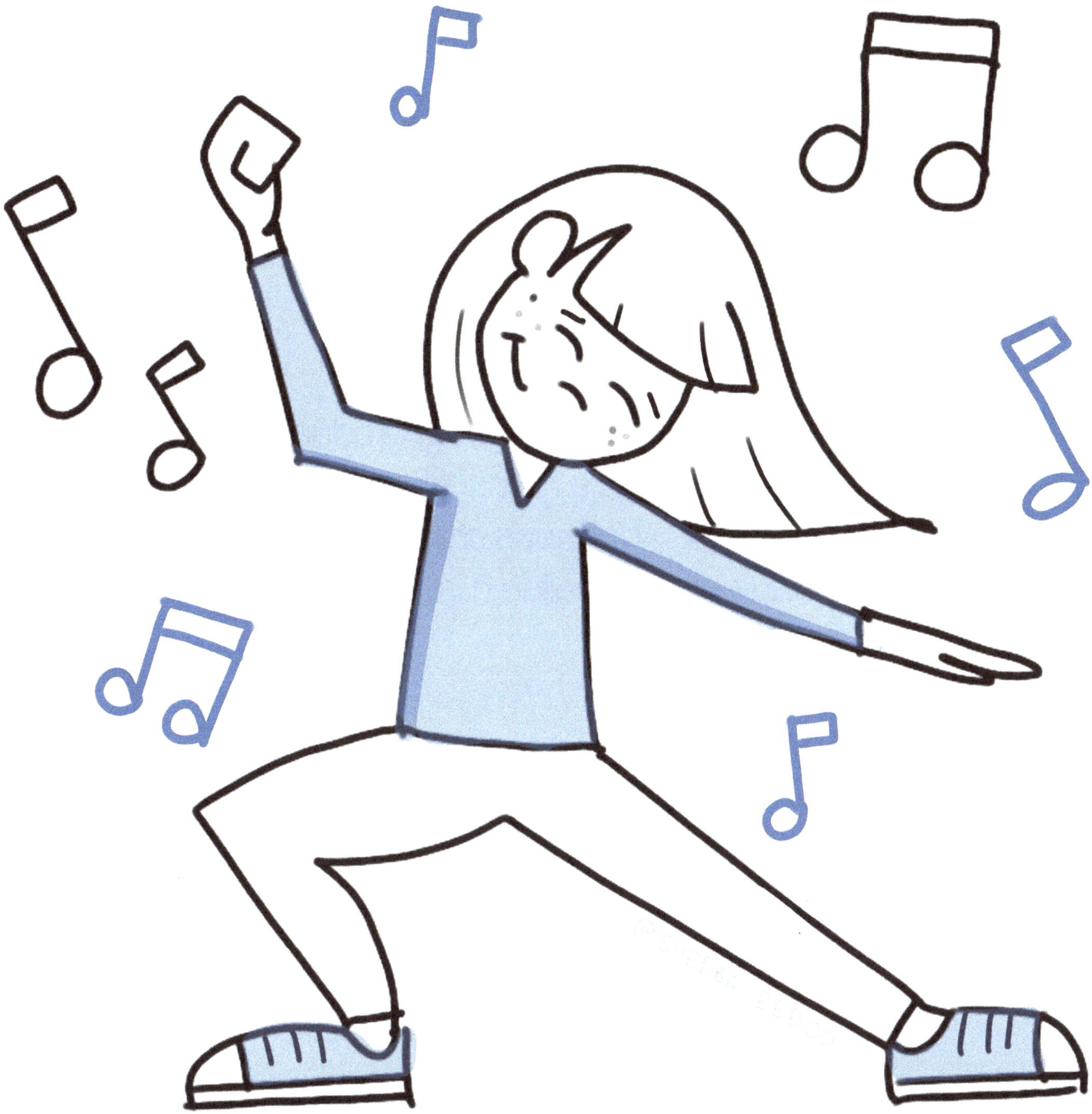

She could try surfing in Hawaii, she could graduate from High School and get her motorcycle license. She started to realize I'm going to be ok and can do most things. She realized she loved to go fast and any adrenaline rush people were scared of she wasn't bothered to try.

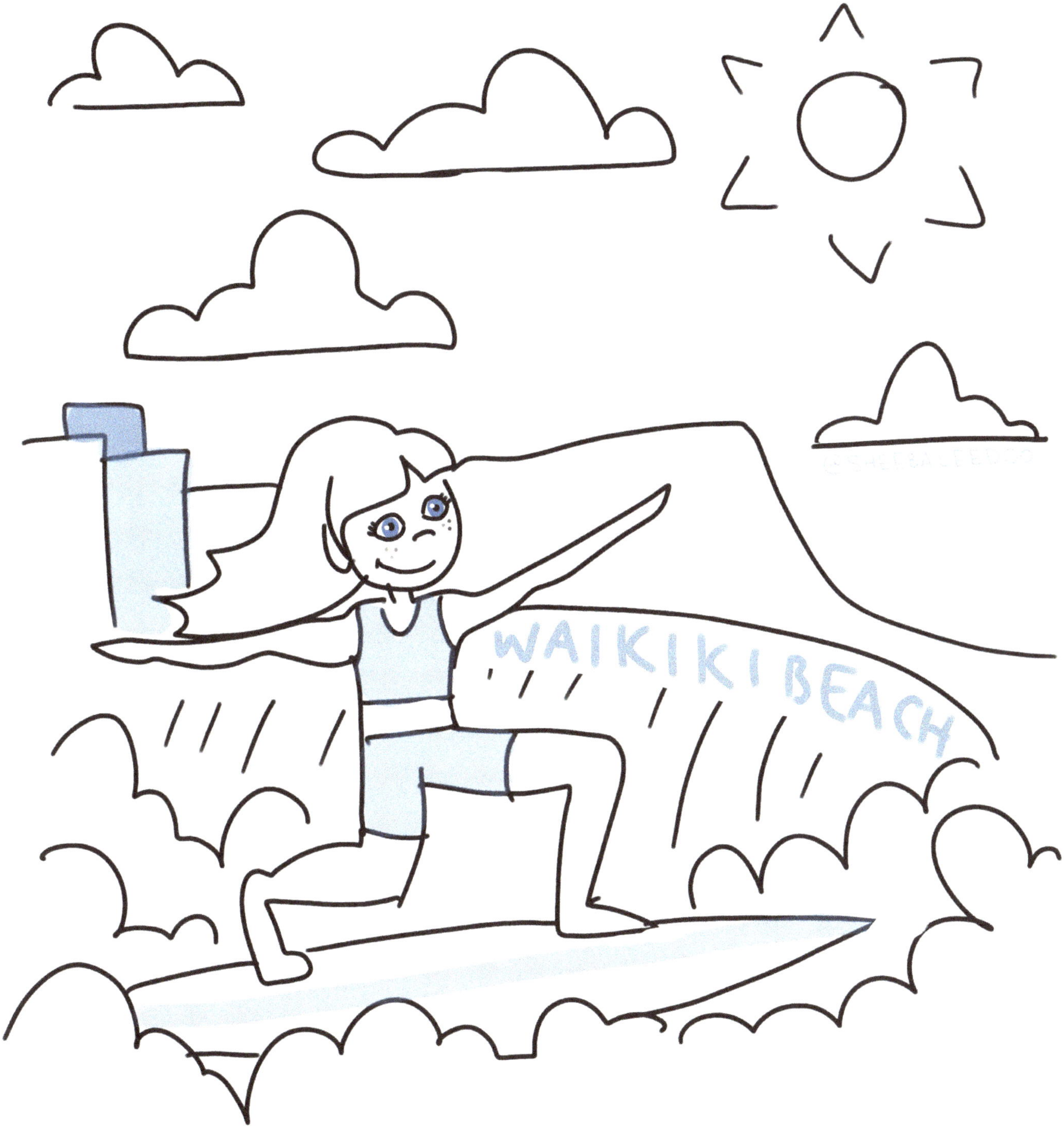
WAIKIKI BEACH

Her Dad would teach her how to drive cars, boats, motorcycles and hunter safety. She was able to obtain her driver's, hunting, boating and motorcycle licenses. She worked hard and followed all the rules set by her state and doctors office.

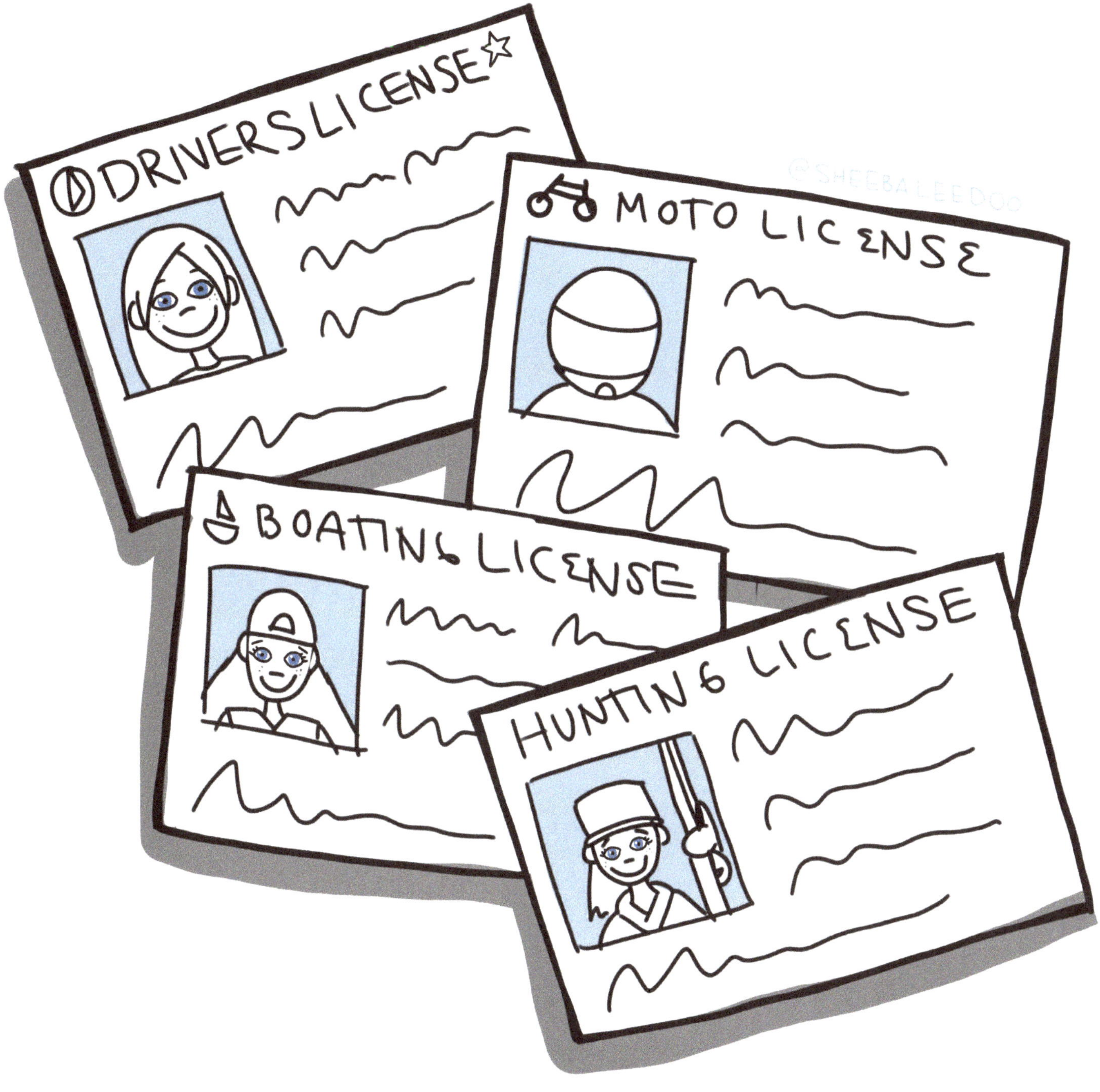
DRIVERS LICENSE
MOTO LICENSE
BOATING LICENSE
HUNTING LICENSE
@SHEEBALEEDOO

She could graduate college while working two jobs. Then she would go into the medical field working with amazing providers. Started in internal medicine for 1 year after graduating college.

Realizing she was interested in Dermatology and wanted to learn more. That would start her Dermatology journey.

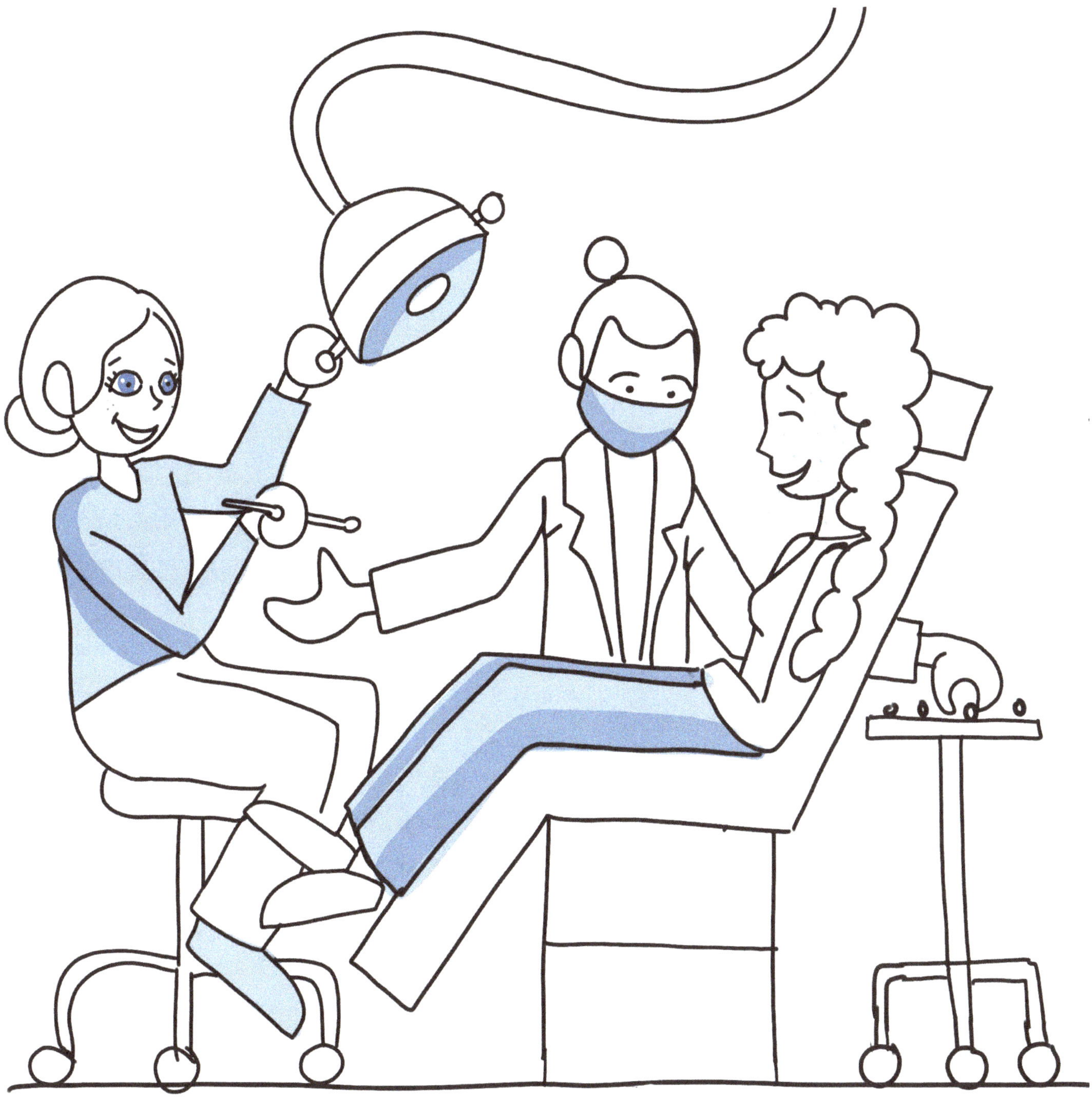

She then continued with Dermatology for almost 18 years. During this time she would help raise her two stepsons since the age 5 and 8. Her family would also include her godchildren's by her side through all their milestones.

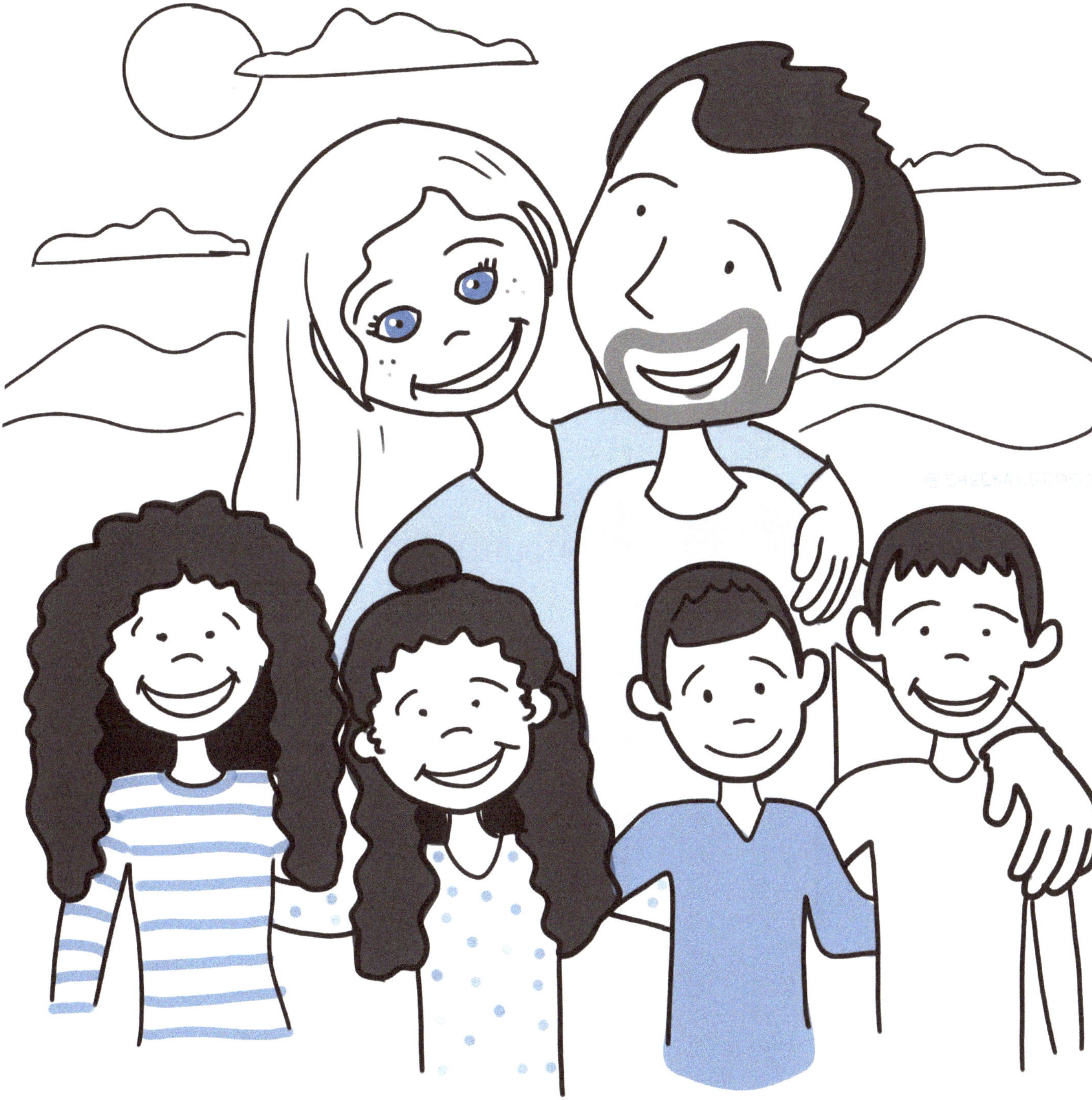

Then she went on to marry her longterm boyfriend. She would continue to live and grow together in this journey of life. This voice would still continuously ask in her head, what else could I do?

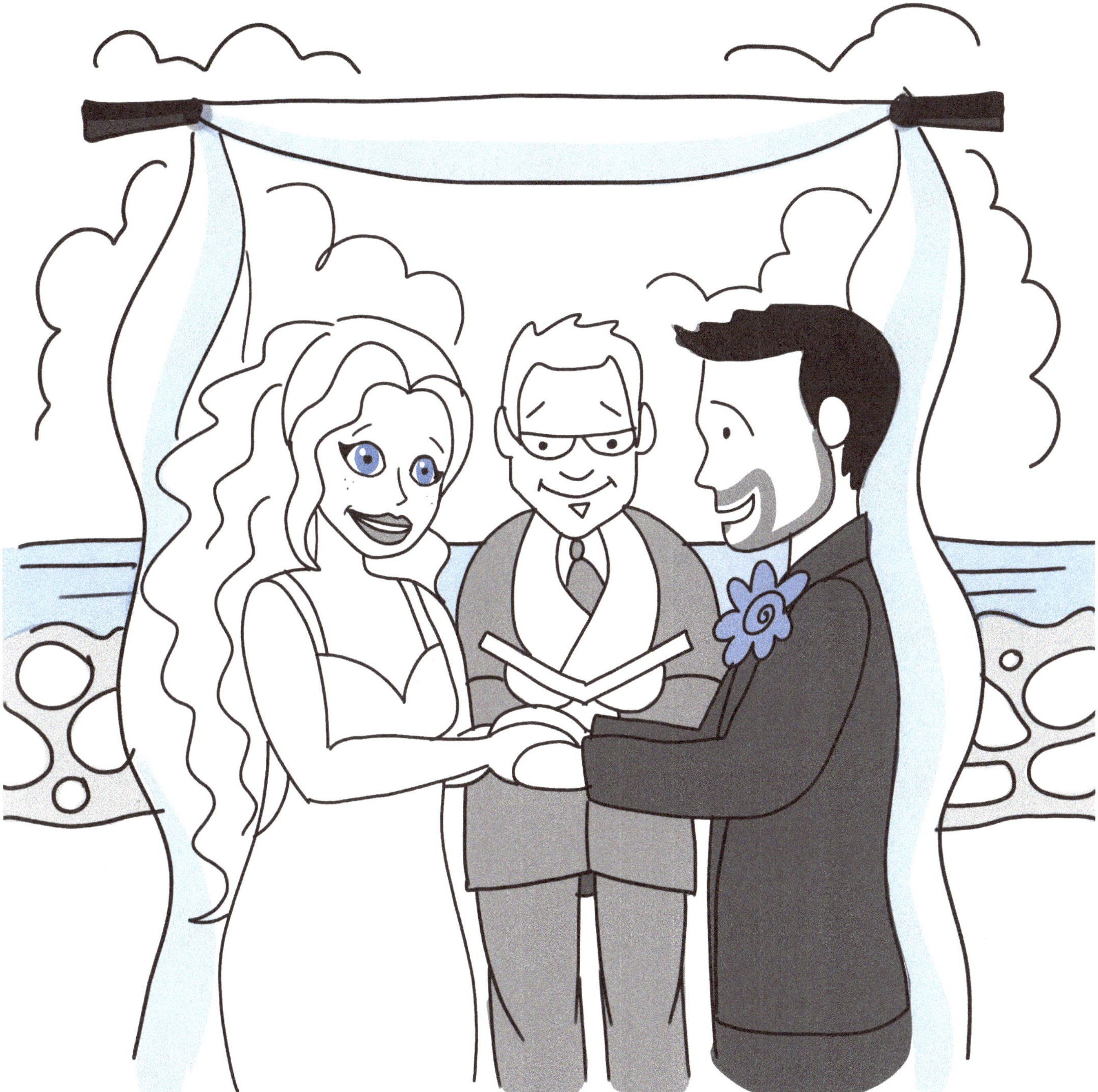

She would end up owning and driving 4 different motorcycles over the years. Her and her husband now have a boat and two jets skis. She still dreams about her next motorcycle. She has learned and continued to apply "what else can I do" to her daily living.

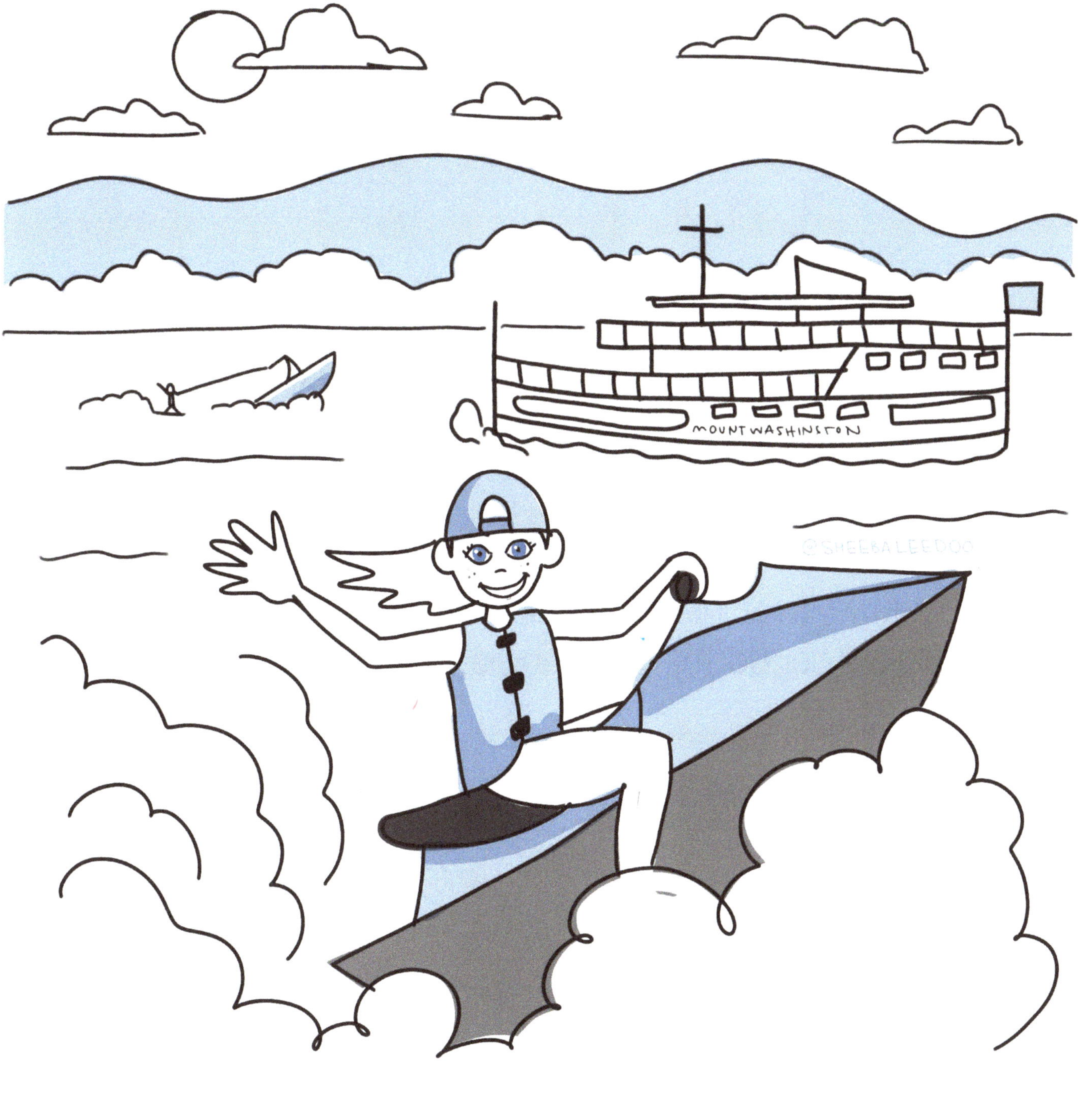
MOUNT WASHINGTON
@SHEEBALEEDOO

Not assuming you can't do it rather can I adapt or change to make this an option. She would tell any child diagnosed with epilepsy now. To encourage them they can still do most things and don't be afraid to ask how.

If she could whisper into her younger selfs ear now as an adult. She would tell her you're going to be ok.

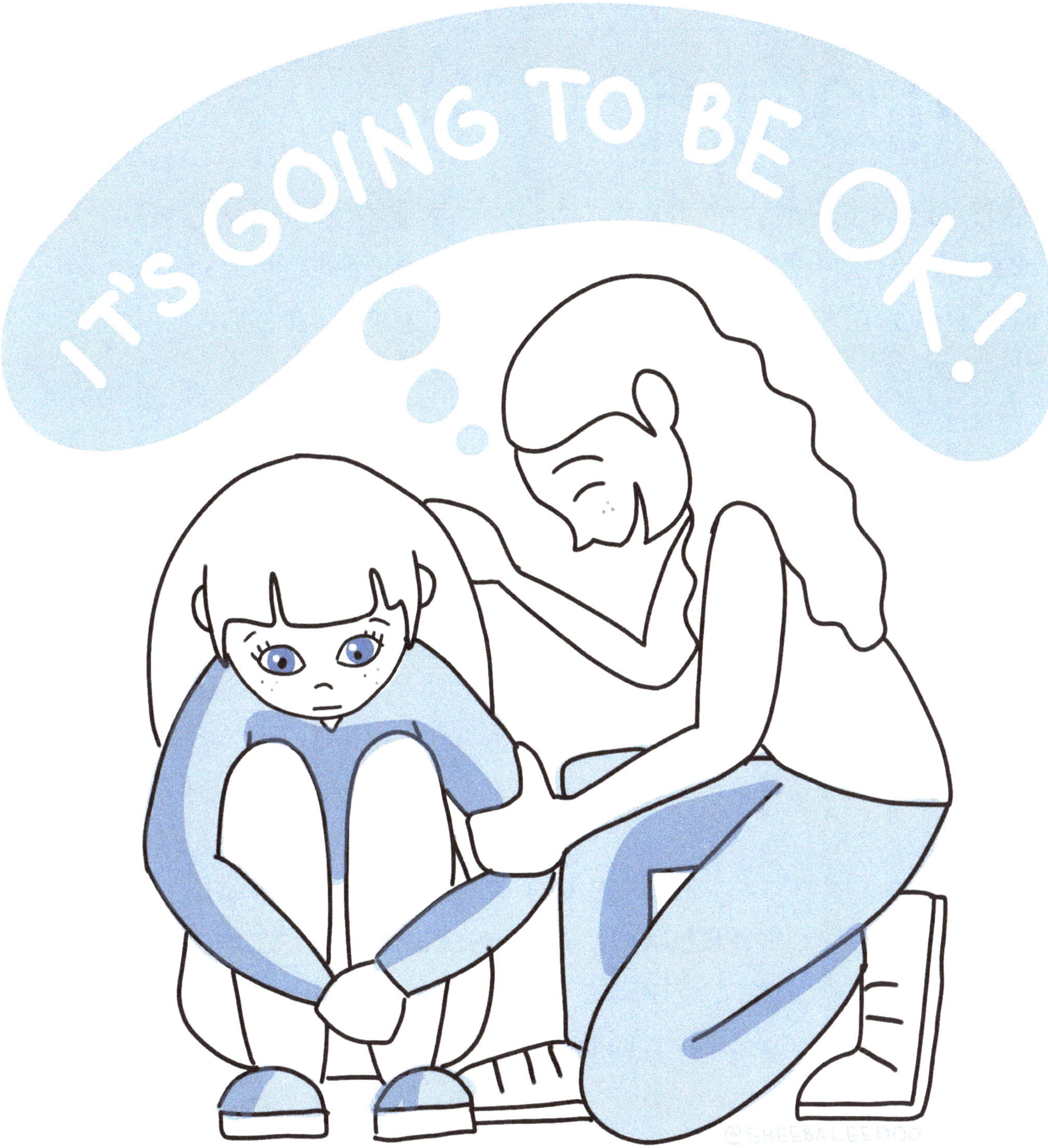
IT'S GOING TO BE OK!
@SHEEBALEEDOO

EPILOGUE

This book was written fueled by being diagnosed with epilepsy and years of living with it. My goal is to help other children no matter where in the journey they are it's going to be ok.

When I was first diagnosed in a little over one month I gained at least 50 pounds after being placed on medication. As an adult it's easier to hide weight and less likely to be questioned. Unfortunately at 13 years of age kids are very honest and not afraid to speak whats on their mind even if it's hurtful. It wasn't uncommon for me to get bullied on the bus daily on my way to school.

It was these comments that would lead me to believe I looked smaller in size if I wore overalls. Hence the title of the book. Most importantly to be kind to everyone as they have a journey you know nothing about.

www.ingramcontent.com/pod-product-compliance
Lightning Source LLC
LaVergne TN
LVHW060046210926
848481LV00013B/3969
* 9 7 9 8 2 1 8 6 1 9 9 1 6 *